CHRONIC LYMPHOCYTIC LEUKEMIA

ESSENTIALS, INSIGHTS AND PARADIGM SHIFTS

DR. BHRATRI BHUSHAN
MBBS, MD, DM
CONSULTANT MEDICAL ONCOLOGY
AND HEMATOLOGY

CONTENTS

In the loving memory
of late Mr. Sunda Ram
(1901-1976).

PREFACE

C hronic lymphocytic leukemia (CLL) is the most common form of leukemia in the western world, although being significantly less common in Asia and Africa. Momentous progress has been made in every aspect of CLL management; from diagnosis, criteria of initiation of treatment, risk stratification, monitoring and treatment.

With increasing understanding of the disease biology, recently there has been an exponential development in the armamentarium of the therapies available and many new drugs have come to the fore and have replaced many conventionally used strategies for the better.

CHAPTER 1: EPIDEMIOLOGY AND ETIOLOGY

C LL (SLL as well) is characterized by un-controlled proliferation of "monoclonal" mature B lymphocytes. The key word here is: Monoclonal. It is the most common leukemia in the western world, constituting about one-third of all leukemias. But it is significantly less common in Asia, while being somewhere in the middle in the African continent. GLOBOCAN estimated worldwide incidence of overall leukemia in 2012 to be 351,965 cases (ASR of 4.7 per 100,000). The incidence of overall leukemia in more developed regions in 2012 was estimated as 141,274 (ASR of 7.2 per 100,000) versus an incidence of 210,691 (3.8 per 100,000 person-years) in less developed regions. GLOBOCAN does not provide specific information about chronic lymphocytic leukemia (CLL).

A US study published in 2004 estimated the worldwide incidence of CLL to be between < 1 and 5.5 per 100,000 people. The highest incidence rates in

2004 were found to be in Australia, US, Ireland and Italy. The US study proposed that CLL is more common in adult males than in females and that CLL presents in caucasians more often than in African-Americans. According to the same study, the median age of diagnosis is between 64 to 70 years, while the German study estimates median age of diagnosis to be between 70 to 72 years. In the US in 2004, five-year survival rate was 83% for those <65 years old and 68% for those 65 years old and older.

The median age of diagnosis in the USA, Europe and Australia is approximately 70 years, with about one quarter of patients aged <65 years and approximately 6% less than 50 years. CLL has a male predominance, and males are more likely to have disease progression and require therapy.

Etiology:

There are some factors which have been found to be associated with an increased incidence of CLL, but overall this disease is more linked with inherent genetic factors rather than environmental ones. The genetic risk factors are also not supported by robust data but the evidence is there. In the following paragraphs we will discuss the current knowledge regarding the etiological agents associated with development of CLL.

DR. BHRATRI BHUSHAN

A retrospective morphologic survey (1973-1983) of 146 cases of malignant lymphoma among the Hawaii-Japanese (migrant Japanese and their off-spring) was conducted to determine whether differences in the incidence and cytologic types of malignant lymphoma exist when compared to those of native Japanese (lifetime residents of Japan). The age-adjusted incidence rates for malignant lymphoma among the Hawaii-Japanese were similar to rates for U.S. whites. However, higher rates for follicular centre cell (FCC) lymphoma with a follicular pattern were observed in the Hawaii-Japanese population when compared with rates for native Japanese. On the basis of the cytologic types of the Lukes-Collins classification, non-Hodgkin's lymphomas among the Hawaii-Japanese resembled those of Western countries, rather than those of Japan. B-cell lymphomas predominated (72 per cent), while T-cell types comprised 23 per cent of cases. Follicular centre cell types were encountered most often (59 per cent), and the small cleaved FCC subtype was the most common (30 percent). The high degree of follicularity (29 per cent) was at variance with the consistently low rates reported in Japan. This may be explained, in part, by higher rates of nodal lymphomas among the Hawaii-Japanese. Of the T-cell lymphomas, diffuse large cell types (T-cell immunoblastic sarcoma, T-IBS), often with cytologic pleomorphism, were relatively frequently encountered (16 per cent), and comprised 15 per-cent of non-Hodgkin's lymphomas; this observation necessitates special clinical and epidemiologic consideration in view of the large Japanese migration to Hawaii from HTLV-I endemic regions of southern Japan. No registered cases of non-Hodgkin's lymphoma or of Hodgkin's disease were documented in Hawaii-Japanese subjects under the age of 15 years. The age-adjusted incidence rates for Hodgkin's disease among the Hawaii-Japanese were similar with those of native Japanese. Nodular sclerosis was the most frequent histologic subtype. The difficulty in distinguishing between Hodgkin's disease and non-Hodgkin's lymphoma, particularly when immunologic cell surface markers are not available, is addressed. Low rates for chronic lymphocytic leukemia among the Hawaii-Japanese were confirmed. Not one well-documented case was identified in the 11-year period surveyed. (Yanagihara ET, Blaisdell RK, Hayashi T & Lukes RJ, 1989).

The incidence of chronic lymphocytic leukemia (CLL) is significantly lower in African Americans than whites, but overall survival is inferior. The biological basis for these observations remains unexplored. The hypothesis is that germline genetic predispositions differ between African Americans and whites with CLL and yield inferior clinical outcomes among African Americans. The study examined a discovery cohort of 42 African American CLL patients ascertained at Duke University and found that the risk allele frequency of most single nucleotide polymorphisms known to confer risk of development for CLL is significantly lower among African Americans than whites. They then confirmed these results in a distinct cohort of 68 African American patients ascertained by the CLL Research Consortium. These results provide the first evidence supporting differential genetic risk for CLL between African Americans compared with whites. (Coombs CC, Rassenti LZ, Falchi L, Slager SL, Strom SS, Ferrajoli A, Weinberg JB, Kipps TJ & Lanasa MC, 2012).

In another study, clinical, cytogenetic, and molecular genetic studies were performed to clarify the pathophysiology of Japanese B cell chronic lymphocytic leukaemia (B-CLL), since the incidence of B-CLL in Japan is significantly lower than in western countries. The clinical and laboratory features of 55 Japanese patients with B-CLL in this study did not differ from those of Americans or Europeans with B-CLL. In the chromosome analyses, suitable metaphases with good band quality were obtained from 48 patients (87.2%), of whom 22 patients (45.8%) showed clonal chromosome aberrations and 14 (29.2%) had non-clonal aberrations. Trisomy 12 and abnormalities of 14q and 13q were found in four (18.2%), two (9.1%) and six patients (27.2%), respectively. There were no particular chromosome abnormalities or specific breakpoints in Japanese B-CLL. However, complex karyotype was found in higher incidence than in western countries. In the Southern blot analyses, rearranged band patterns were observed in the major breakpoint region (mbr) of the bcl-2 gene in one case, in the 5'-breakpoint region (5'-bcl-2) in two, and bcl-3 in one. Of the two patients with 5'-bcl-2 rearrangements, one had a normal karyotype and the other had t(2;18)(p12;q21). The incidence of rearrangements of the bcl-1, bcl-2 and bcl-3 genes in Japanese B-CLL was similar to that in western countries. These findings suggest that the biological characteristics of B-CLL in Japan are almost the same as those in western countries, although the incidence of B-CLL in Japan is quite different; this may be related to racial differences, which seem to be an important factor in the development of B-CLL. (Asou H, Takechi M, Tanaka K, Tashiro S, Dohy H, Ohno R & Kamada N, 1993).

The risk of specific histologic types of leukemia among farmers was investigated using mortality records from Nebraska for the years 1957-1974. The frequency of farming as an occupation listed on the death certificates among 1,084 leukemia deaths was compared to the corresponding frequency for 2,168 controls for calculation of odds ratios (OR). The elevated OR for chronic lymphocytic leukemia among farmers was statistically significant (OR = 1.67), while elevated ORs for acute lymphatic leukemia (OR = 1.34), acute monocytic leukemia (OR = 1.94), and acute unspecified leukemia (OR = 2.36) were not. Farmers who died at younger ages or who were born in more recent years were at greater risk of acute lymphatic, acute myeloid, chronic myeloid, acute unspecified, and unspecified leukemia than other farmers. Certain cell types were related to agricultural characteristics of the subject's county of residence, although few were statistically significant. Farmers from counties with large cattle inventories and significant daily activity were at higher risk of chronic lymphocytic leukemia. Farmers from major corn-producing, hog- and chicken-raising, and pesticide- and fertilizer-using counties tended to be at higher risk of acute lymphatic, acute myeloid, chronic myeloid, and acute unspecified leukemia than farmers from counties less involved in the production or use of these agricultural factors. (Blair A & White DW,1985).

Death certificate analyses of 1675 white, male Iowans over age 30 years who died of leukemia in 1964-1978 were completed. Each case was matched to two controls on age (within two years) at death, county of usual residence and year of death. Consideration of usual occupation, as recorded on the death certificate, resulted in an odds ratio for leukemia mortality among farmers of 1.24

(p less than 0.05). The highest odds ratios for farmers were observed in those born after 1890, those dying after 1970, and those dying at age 65 years or younger. Odds ratios for farmers were also elevated in counties with high soybean and corn production per acre for those born between 1890 and 1900. For those born after 1900, odds ratios for farmers were increased in counties with the greatest numbers of egg-laying chickens and largest number of acres treated with herbicides. The types of leukemia causing elevated mortalities in Iowa farmers were chronic lymphatic and unspecified lymphatic. Mortality from unspecified lymphatic leukemia was associated with corn per acre, number of milk cows and number of egg-laying chickens. (Burmeister LF, Van Lier SF & Isacson P, 1982).

Another study assessed the effect of occupational solvent exposure on the risk of adult chronic lymphocytic leukemia (CLL). This case-control study was nested in the Nordic Occupational Cancer Study (NOCCA) cohort. 20,615 CLL cases diagnosed in 1961-2005 in Finland, Iceland, Norway, and Sweden, and 103,075 population-based controls matched by year of birth, sex, and country were included. Occupational histories for cases and controls were obtained from census records in 1960, 1970, 1980/1981, and 1990. Exposure to selected solvents was estimated by using the NOCCA job-exposure matrix (NOCCA-JEM). Odds ratios (OR) and 95% confidence intervals (95% CI) were estimated by using conditional logistic regression models. Overall, nonsignificant CLL risk elevations were observed for methylene chloride, perchloroethylene, and 1,1,1-trichloroethane. Compared to unexposed, significantly increased risks were observed for cumulative perchloroethylene exposure≤13.3 ppm-years (OR = 1.85, 95% CI 1.16-2.96) and average life-time perchloroethylene exposure≤2.5 ppm (1.61, 95% CI 1.01-2.56) among women, and cumulative methylene chloride exposure≤12.5 ppm-years (OR = 1.19, 95% CI 1.01-1.41) and 12.5-74.8 ppm-years (OR = 1.23, 95% CI 1.01-1.51) among menin an analysis with 5 years lag-time, though without dose-response pattern. Decreased CLL risk was observed for aliphatic and alicyclic hydrocarbon solvents and toluene. This study did not support associations for solvent exposure and CLL. Observed weak associations for methylene chloride, perchloroethylene, 1,1,1-trichloroethane exposures, aliphatic and alicyclic hydrocarbons and toluene were not consistent across sexes, and showed no gradient with amount of exposure. (Talibov M, Auvinen A, Weiderpass E, Hansen J, Martinsen JI, Kjaerheim K, Tryggvadottir L & Pukkala E, 2017).

A group of researchers did an analysis of data on the incidence of leukemia, lymphoma and myeloma in the Life Span Study cohort of atomic bomb survivors during the period from late 1950 through the end of 1987 (93,696 survivors accounting for 2,778,000 person-years). These analyses added 9 additional years of follow-up for leukemia and 12 for myeloma to that in the last comprehensive reports on these diseases. This was the first analysis of the lymphoma incidence data in the cohort. Using both the Leukemia Registry and the Hiroshima and Nagasaki tumor registries, a total of 290 leukemia, 229 lymphoma and 73 myeloma cases were identified. The primary analyses were restricted to first primary tumors diagnosed among residents of the cities or surrounding areas with Dosimetry System 1986 dose estimates between 0 and 4 Gy kerma (231 leukemias, 208 lymphomas and 62 myelomas). Analyses focused on time-dependent models for the excess absolute risk. Separate analyses were carried out for acute lymphocytic leukemia (ALL), acute myelogenous leukemia (AML), chronic myelocytic leukemia (CML) and adult T-cell leukemia (ATL). There were few cases of chronic lymphocytic leukemia in this population. There was strong evidence of radiation-induced risks for all subtypes except ATL, and there were significant subtype differences with respect to the effects of age at exposure and sex and in the temporal pattern of risk. The AML dose-response function was nonlinear, whereas there was no evidence against linearity for the other subtypes. When averaged over the follow-up period, the excess absolute risk (EAR) estimates (in cases per 10(4) PY Sv) for the leukemia subtypes were 0.6, 1.1 and 0.9 for ALL, AML and CML, respectively. The corresponding estimated average excess relative risks at 1 Sv are 9.1, 3.3 and 6.2 respectively. There was some evidence of an increased risk of lymphoma in males (EAR = 0.6 cases per 10(4) PY Sv) but no evidence of any excess in females. There was no evidence of an excess risk for multiple myeloma in our standard analyses. (Preston DL, Kusumi S, Tomonaga M, Izumi S, Ron E, Kuramoto A, Kamada N, Dohy H, Matsuo T & Matsuo T,1994).

Investigations on the association between environmental hazards and the development of various types of leukaemia were reviewed in an analysis. Regarding acute non-lymphocytic leukaemia (ANLL) exposure to ionizing radiation is a well-documented risk factor. According to several studies exposure to strong electromagnetic fields may be suspected to be of etiologic importance for ANLL. There is evidence that occupational handling of benzene is a risk factor and other organic solvents may also be leukemogenic. Occupational exposure to petrol products has been proposed to be a risk factor although the hazardous substances have not yet been defined. Results of cytogenetic studies in ANLL suggest that exposure to certain environmental agents may be associated with relatively specific clonal chromosome aberrations. These results are of interest because it has been proposed that chromosomal rearrangements may play a role in the activation of cellular oncogenes. Exposure in utero to ionizing radiation has been proposed to be a risk factor for acute lymphocytic leukaemia (ALL) in children. Unlike ANLL there seems at present to be little evidence that ALL is related to exposure to some chemicals. Chronic myeloid leukaemia (CML) may follow exposure to high doses of ionizing radiation whereas such exposure seems to be of insignificant importance for the development of chronic lymphocytic leukaemia (CLL). According to some studies an abnormally high incidence of CLL may be found among farmers in the USA. These results have not been confirmed in Scandinavian studies. There seems to be little evidence that CML or CLL are related to occupational handling of some chemicals. (Brandt L, 1985).

Increasing evidence points to a heritable contribution in the development of lymphoma. A study was done to determine the rate of familial lymphoproliferative malignancy among consecutive lymphoma patients presenting to a tertiary care center and to enroll families with multiple affected first-degree relatives on a data and tissue collection study. Beginning in 2004 all new patients presenting to the Dana-Farber Cancer Institute with non-Hodgkin (NHL) or Hodgkin lymphoma (HL) or chronic lymphocytic leukaemia (CLL) were asked to complete a one-page self-administered family history questionnaire. 55.4% of 1948 evaluable patients reported a first-degree relative with a malignancy, with the highest rate among CLL probands. Lymphoid malignancies were particularly common, with 9.4% of all probands reporting a first-degree relative with a related lymphoproliferative disorder (LPD). This frequency was again highest for CLL, at 13.3% of CLL probands, compared to 8.8% of NHL probands and 5.9% of HL probands (P = 0.002). The prevalence of CLL was significantly increased in parents of CLL probands (P<0.05), and a greater risk of NHL was seen in fathers of NHL probands than in mothers (P = 0.026). We conclude that familial aggregation of LPDs is common among newly diagnosed patients, varies significantly by diagnosis and contributes meaningfully to the population disease burden. (Brown JR, Neuberg D, Phillips K, Reynolds H, Silverstein J, Clark JC, Ash M, Thompson C, Fisher DC, Jacobsen E, LaCasce AS & Freedman AS, 2008).

Monoclonal B-cell lymphocytosis (MBL) is an asymptomatic haematological condition characterized by low absolute levels of B-cell clones with a surface immunophenotype similar to that of chronic lymphocytic leukaemia (CLL). In the general population, MBL increases with age with a prevalence of 5-9% in individuals over age 60 years. It has been reported to be higher among first-degree relatives from CLL families. We report results of multi-parameter flow cytometry among 505 first-degree relatives with no personal history of lymphoproliferative disease from 140 families having at least two cases of CLL. Seventeen percent of relatives had MBL. Age was the most important determinant where the probability for developing MBL by age 90 years was 61%. MBL clustered in certain families but clustering was independent of the number of known CLL cases in a family. As is the case with CLL, males had a significantly higher risk for MBL than did females (P = 0·04). MBL patients had significantly higher mean absolute lymphocyte counts (2·4×10(9) /l) and B-cell counts (0·53×10(9) /l) than those with a normal B-cell immuno-phenotype. Our findings show that MBL occurs at a very high rate in high risk CLL families. Both the age and gender distribution of MBL are parallel to CLL, implying a shared inherited risk. (Goldin LR, Lanasa MC, Slager SL, Cerhan JR, Vachon CM, Strom SS, Camp NJ, Spector LG, Leis JF, Morrison VA, Glenn M, Rabe KG, Achenbach SJ, Algood SD, Abbasi F, Fontaine L, Yau M, Rassenti LZ, Kay NE, Call TG, Hanson CA, Weinberg JB, Marti GE & Caporaso NE, 2010).

With the advent and increased availability of advanced techniques for studying genome at a deeper level, many new insights are being unravelled at a prolific pace but nothing conclusively could be said at the present moment and translation of whatever association that have been found till date in to clinical practice is inherently problematic.

CHAPTER 2: DIAGNOSIS

Symptoms:
The clinical presentations of a patient of CLL are heterogeneous. While most of the patients are discovered incidentally, meaning that they just don't have any symptoms or signs suggestive of any disease and the workup done as a routine reveals lymphocytosis; some patients may present with enlargement of lymph nodes. A minority of the patients present with "B" symptoms, which are: unintentional weight loss ≥10 percent of body weight within the previous six months, fever of >100.5°F (>38°C) for ≥2 weeks without evidence of infection, drenching night sweats without evidence of infection and extreme fatigue. Rarely, patients may present with features such as auto-immune hemolytic anemia, thrombocytopenia, PRCA, frequent infections that signify an immuno-deficiency state and a peculiar hypersensitivity to insect bites. In some cases of extreme lymphocytosis neurological symptoms like stroke or TIA may be present. It is important to remember that most patients don't have any symptoms at presentation

and it comes quite as a shock for the patient to learn about his diagnosis.

Signs:

A characteristic type of lymphadenopathy is the most common physical sign present in patients of CLL, that can be seen in more than half of the patients but the degree of lymph node enlargement and the numbers of lymph nodes involved vary greatly among patients. The affected nodes are firm, rounded, discrete, nontender, and freely mobile upon palpation. Most often lymph nodes above the diaphragm are affected, although lymph nodes of any region may be involved. Spleen is also frequently enlarged in many patients, in some patients, disease of whom has been left unattended, it could be quite massive and may create confusion regarding the primary diagnosis.

Skin is the most commonly affected extra lymphoid organ. Leukaemia cutis is seen in very few patients. Skin manifestations may also be result of the disturbances caused by manifestations of CLL, like thrombocytopenia may give rise to purpura and infections may set in due to immunodeficiency.

Other organs like liver, kidneys, meninges and intestines may be affected rarely but their involvement is not a characteristic feature of CLL and if these are predominantly involved then other lymphoma are more frequently found to be blamed.

Tests:

The International Workshop on Chronic Lympho-cytic Leukemia (iwCLL) has proposed many criteria virtually covering all aspects of CLL management, ranging from diagnosis to response assessment. In the past there were other criteria as well, but now-adays iwCLL criteria are universally accepted and followed.

The World Health Organization classification of hematopoietic neoplasias describes CLL as leu-kemic, lymphocytic lymphoma, being only dis-tinguishable from small lymphocytic lymphoma (SLL) by its leukemic manifestation. It is important to note here that these diagnosis pertain to dis-ease arising from only B-cell clones, not by T-cells, which are a different entity. Sometimes morph-ology is not enough to differentiate CLL from other neoplasms of B-cells and even if the microscopic picture is characteristic, other tests like immuno-phenotyping and genetic studies have to be done to formulate a proper treatment plan according to the body of science that has been validated and practiced. (Michael Hallek, Bruce D. Cheson, Dan-iel Catovsky, Federico Caligaris-Cappio, Guillermo

Dighiero, Hartmut Döhner, Peter Hillmen, Michael Keating, Emili Montserrat, Nicholas Chiorazzi, Stephan Stilgenbauer, Kanti R. Rai, John C. Byrd, Barbara Eichhorst, Susan O'Brien, Tadeusz Robak, John F. Seymour and Thomas J. Kipps, 2018).

Peripheral blood features:

The diagnosis of CLL requires the presence of ≥ 5 $\times 10^{9}$/L B lymphocytes in the peripheral blood, sustained for at least 3 months. The clonality of these B lymphocytes needs to be confirmed by demonstrating immunoglobulin light chain restriction using flow cytometry. Morphologically these cells are characteristically small, mature lymphocytes with a narrow rim of cytoplasm and a dense nucleus lacking discernable nucleoli. Smudge cells are a common finding.

Sometimes larger cells are seen along with characteristic small lymphocytes, these are known as prolymphocytes and if their percentage is 55 or more then the diagnosis is prolymphocytic leukemia (PLL) which is virtually identical to CLL by immunophenotyping but has a worse prognosis in comparison.

In presence of lymphadenopathy, splenomegaly, hepatomegaly, anemia, thrombocytopenia and/or symptoms (vide infra), a diagnosis of CLL or SLL could be made even in the monoclonal B lymphocytes are <5000/microL. And if none of these features are present then these cases with below threshold monoclonal B lymphocytes population are known as monoclonal B lymphocytosis (MBL). MBL may progress to CLL at a rate of 1 to 2 % per year.

When peripheral blood shows monoclonal B lymphocytes <5000/microL **and** there is lymphadenopathy which upon histological examination shows involvement with these cells but **without** anemia and/or thrombocytopenia, the diagnosis is SLL. Although it is not advisable to do a lymph node biopsy of an unsuspicious lymph node in a patient who incidentally shows monoclonal B lymphocytes <5000/microL, just to see whether or not SLL **may be** present; such cases should be labelled as MBL.

Immunophenotyping:

The most important role that immunophenotyping plays is to establish the clonality of B cells, which is ascertained by restriction to expression of either κ or λ immunoglobulin light chain, **never both.** CD5 is very useful in making a diagnosis of CLL, along with positivity of CD23 and CD19, but it's important to remember that CD5 is not exclusive of other malignancies. The levels of sIg CD20 (as well as CD79b) is characteristically low (dim). In most of the cases, a diagnosis can be reached by using these markers and if not then others are there, but their usefulness is uncertain. A consensus "recommended" panel of such markers to refine diagnosis in borderline cases (CD43, CD79b, CD81, CD200, CD10, and ROR1) has been defined. (Andy C. Rawstrone et al., 2017)

Genetic studies:

Deletions of the long arm of chromosome 13 is the most common abnormality found on interphase FISH (fluorescence in situ hybridization) on peripheral blood, others are *trisomy* of chromosome 12, *deletion* of the long arm of chromosome 11 and *deletion* of the short arm of chromosome 17. Such findings are found in the majority of CLL patients. Conventional metaphase karyotyping coupled with the aforementioned interphase FISH studies may not only help to make a diagnosis of CLL (it must be noted that these are **not required to make a diagnosis of CLL**) and obtain additional prognostic information but also in identifying other malignancies that have characteristic chromosomal abnormalities.

The main utility of these tests lies in decision making regarding treatment selection. It has been validated in trials that del(17p) and/or *TP53* mutations (as determined by DNA sequencing, with a cutoff of 10%) confer poor prognosis overall. These patients fare especially poorly on conventional chemo-immunotherapy protocols and BTK inhibitors or BCL2 targeting drugs are better options. So it is essential to know whether or not the patients had del(17p) or TP53 mutation (**both** ought to be studied).

Patients with del (11q) or trisomy 12 also have a poorer prognosis compared with those with normal karyotype (found in less than 20% of the patients) or those with del (13q). NGS has shed light upon other abnormalities like NOTCH1 and SF3B1 but they are not yet a part of routine evaluation.

Immunoglobulin heavy chain:

When the sequencing of leukemia cells' immunoglobulin variable heavy chain gene shows an **unmutated** (98% homology) status, it is an **unfavorable** prognostic marker. On the other hand, mutated status is favorable and predictive of a good response to FCR regimen. Interestingly, ZAP-70 and CD38 (which are immunophenotypic markers) show correlation (which is not absolute) with **unmutated** IGHV, thus imparting poor prognosis.

Bone marrow examination:

It is important to clarify that in the present era of immunophenotyping and molecular genetics, bone marrow examination is **not needed for establishing a diagnosis.** That being said, in certain situations it is necessary. Like in determining whether the persistent cytopenia is due to leukemic infiltration of the bone marrow or due to the effects of therapy. Also, it is **required** to declare the response to therapy being complete (CR).

Apart from these studies, that are directed towards the diagnosis of CLL; physical examination, routine blood chemistry, direct antiglobulin (Coombs) test (being positive in upto 35% cases, but leading to AIHA in a minority), HIV, hepatitis B, hepatitis C, CMV (in select cases) testing, serum immunoglobulin levels, chest X-ray/CT scanning, CT scanning of other areas of interest (ultrasound in resource poor settings) are also to be done. PET-CT is **not** recommended.

CHAPTER 3: INDICATIONS FOR TREATMENT

E ach and every patient of CLL doesn't require treatment. Those with Rai stage 0 derive no benefit regarding survival outcomes by early initiation of treatment and while treatment may be contemplated in Rai stage one and two for other reasons, survival outcomes remain the same despite beginning early treatment nevertheless. So in Rai stage zero, one and two observation alone suffices in the majority of the patients. In these patients of low and intermediate risk according to the Rai classification, treatment may be indicated based on other factors, which we will discuss subsequently.

Patients who belong to the high risk Rai group, i.e stage three and four, require treatment as without therapy they will succumb to the disease process. The international workshop on CLL criteria elaborate the decision making regarding patients selection. These are universally followed and are briefly discussed here. The disease is said to be "active" if any **one** (or more) criteria is fulfilled.

1. Presence or development of anemia (Hb less than 10 g/dl) or platelet count less than 100,000/microL.
2. Splenomegaly which is symptomatic or progressive or more than 6 cm below costal margin
3. Lymph node enlargement which is symptomatic or progressive of more than 10 cm in longest diameter
4. Progressive lymphocytosis with an increase of ≥50% over a 2-month period, or lymphocyte doubling time (LDT) <6 months.
5. Unresponsive autoimmune anemia or thrombocytopenia
6. Extranodal involvement
7. Disease-related symptoms as defined by any of the following:
    1. Unintentional weight loss ≥10% within the previous 6 months.
    2. ECOG performance scale 2 or worse
    3. Fevers ≥100.5°F or 38.0°C for 2 or more weeks without evidence of infection.
    4. Night sweats for ≥1 month without evidence of infection.

It is important to note here that lymphocyte count at presentation, no matter how high, is not an indication of treatment. Treatment may be initiated in some patients of high lymphocyte count if clinical features mandate but the decision should be individualised.

These criteria apply to relapsed or refractory (R/R) disease as well. It sounds a little counterintuitive for the uninitiated but some patients of R/R CLL may live long without any treatment based on the aforementioned criteria.

CHAPTER 4: STAGING

The staging systems used in CLL are based on physical examination and elementary blood work, without any necessity to perform radiological studies. These are called Rai and Binet staging systems and are accepted worldwide, both for patient management and clinical trials. These systems assist in prognostication and decision making regarding whether or not therapy should be started.

Rai staging system:

According to this system patients of CLL are classified in three groups:

1. Low-risk disease: patients who have lymphocytosis with leukemia cells in the blood and/or marrow (formerly considered Rai stage 0).
2. Patients with peripheral blood lymphocytosis, enlarged lymph nodes in any site, and splenomegaly and/or hepatomegaly (lymph nodes being palpable or not) are

defined as having intermediate-risk disease (formerly considered Rai stage I or II).

3. High-risk disease includes patients with disease-related anemia (as defined by a hemoglobin [Hb] level < 11 g/dL) (formerly stage III) or thrombocytopenia (as defined by a platelet count of <100 × 10^9/L; formerly stage IV).

(KR Rai, A Sawitsky, EP Cronkite, AD Chanana, RN Levy & BS Pasternack, 1975)

It is important to note here that in Rai system consideration is given only to the presence or absence of enlargement of lymph nodes rather than numbers of involved lymph node areas, assessment of which is a feature of Binet system.

The prognostic information in the original series for: stage 0, is greater than 150; stage I 101; stage II, 71; stage III, 19; stage IV, 19, The median survival for the entire series was 71 months.

Binet staging system:

The Binet staging system is based on the number of involved lymphoid areas, as defined by the presence of enlarged lymph nodes ≥1 cm in diameter or organomegaly, and on whether there is anemia or thrombocytopenia.

Areas of involvement considered for staging include:

1. Head and neck, including the Waldeyer ring (this counts as 1 area, even if ≥1 group of nodes is enlarged).
2. Axillae (involvement of both axillae counts as just 1 area).
3. Groins, including superficial femorals (involvement of both groins counts as just 1 area).
4. Palpable spleen.
5. Palpable liver (clinically enlarged).

Stage A. Hb ≥10 g/dL and platelets ≥100 × 10^9/L and up to 2 of these areas involved.

Stage B. Hb ≥10 g/dL and platelets ≥100 × 10^9/L and 3 or more of the lymphoid areas involved.

Stage C. Hb <10 g/dL and/or a platelet count <100 × 10^9/L.

(Professor J. L. Binet, A. Auquier, G. Dighiero, C. Chastang, H. Piguet, J. Goasguen, G. Vaugier, G. Potron, P. Colona, F. Oberling, M. Thomas, G. Tchernia, C. Jacquillat, P. Boivin, C. Lesty, M. T. Duault, M. Monconduit, S. Belabbes & F. Gremy, 1981)

As far as staging models are concerned, these two are the most widely used ones but as is evident from our discussion, these are not reflective of the progress that has recently been made in understanding of the biology of the disease. In the first chapter, we have discussed about the contribution of molecular genetics in prognostication and therapeutic decision making.

Many models have been proposed to incorporate this information, and some of them have been validated but the most commonly used model is the CLL-IPI (CLL international prognostic index).

CLL International Prognostic Index (2016)

	Adverse Factor	Grade
Age	>65 years	1
Clinical Stage	Rai I-IV or Binet B-C	1
β_2-microglobulin level	>3.5 mg/L	2
IGHV mutation status	Unmutated (>98% homology with germline)	2
Del(17p) and/or TP53 mutation	Present	4

Risk	Score	5-year Overall Survival (p<0.001 for all)
Low	0-1	93%
Intermediate	2-3	79%
High	4-6	63%
Very High	7-10	23%

CLL-IPI is a great tool for prognostication and it further refines the Rai and Binet systems. Overall, the most important risk defining characteristic is deletion of the short arm of chromosome 17 and/or TP53 mutation. The latter has clear implications on selection of therapy both in the first and subsequent lines; although now IGHV mutation status in also coming to the fore in therapeutic decision making.

CHAPTER 5: FIRST LINE TREATMENT

It should be stressed that there is no single "gold standard" treatment approach that one can choose freely over others. There are options available more than ever before and newer drugs and their combinations are translating into clinical benefits. At present for the first line therapy in CLL patients, the available drugs are: venetoclax, ibrutinib, rituximab (R), ofatumumab, obinutuzumab, fludarabine (F), pentostatin (P), bendamustine (B), chlorambucil and cyclophosphamide (C). Various combinations of these drugs are approved as initial therapies and each has its unique challenges and particular situations where one drug is better than others. But it's difficult to make generalisations.

That being said, guidelines and expert recommendations are there to help in clinical decision making. The first dichotomy is whether the patient is young or elderly. The distinction is not clear and a somewhat rigid frame of age less than 70 years and

70 years or more is resorted to. There may be exceptions if the clinician feels that the physiological age seems discordant with the chronological age. And the second important deciding factor (maybe even more important than age) is deletion 17p or TP53 mutation status.

We can classify the patients for the purpose of treatment selection in the following way:

1. Patients **without** deletion 17p/*TP53* mutation and IGHV-**unmutated** (further divided into young or elderly)
2. Patients **without** deletion 17p/*TP53* mutation and IGHV-**mutated** (further divided into young or elderly)
3. Patients **with** deletion 17p/*TP53* mutation **regardless** of IGHV status (**regardless** of age)

Young patients:

Previously, in young patients (<70 years of age) combination chemoimmunotherapy, FCR, was an obvious choice. Lately, in a subset of these patients who have IGHV-**un**mutated status **without** deletion 17p or TP53 mutation, ibrutinib with/without rituximab has become the preferred choice.

The data supporting this approach come from the

phase III ECOG-ACRIN E1912 trial. This trial compared ibrutinib plus rituximab against FCR in young patients **with** IGHV-**un**mutated status **without** deletion 17p. Although not all patients were tested for IGHV mutation status. The former combination resulted in improved PFS, OS and decreased toxicity.

The survival benefits are clearly there for ibrutinib +/- rituximab, but the problem is that the time duration of taking ibrutinib is indefinite, warranting a virtually lifelong dependence on this costly drug, cost being an ever more important issue in resource poor settings.

Young patients who have IGHV-mutation **but not** deletion 17p/TP53 mutation, have a choice between ibrutinib (+/- rituximab) and FCR. There are pros and cons of both; in my opinion if patients of such a profile are fit enough to tolerate combined chemoimmunotherapy then FCR is a better option. FCR not only provides good PFS and OS benefits, but also has the potential of delivering long-term cure. Yet, it can't be stressed enough that it's very toxic and morbidity and mortality risks must be reckoned with.

Other commonly opted options are combination of fludarabine and rituximab (FR), fludarabine and cyclophosphamide (FC) and rituximab plus bendamustine (BR). There are other options as well like adding mitoxantrone to FCR (R-FCM) and pentostatin based combinations. Out of these options FCR is the best as far as overall disease control and thus attainment of survival outcomes is concerned but it very toxic and a vast number of patients were unable to finish the prescribed treatment cycles in the studies. In practice too, we often find toxicities like myelosuppression and resultant infection prohibitive and sometimes fatal. FR is a somewhat less toxic and almost equally efficacious alternative, but as the clinical situation of is, if a patient is thought to be fit enough to tolerate FR then FCR would also be well tolerated, thus making it hard to select a target population for this combination. BR is not commonly used in younger patients, whereas in older patients it's a good option. Combinations like R-FCM add unnecessary toxicity to an already very toxic regimen and in my opinion should be avoided. Pentostatin based combination chemo-immunotherapy is used too, albeit less widely than fludarabine based ones.

Now coming to patients **with** deletion 17p or TP53 mutation, treatment selection has been most refined in this subset. Regardless of the age of the patient, ibrutinib or venetoclax plus obinutuzumab are the preferred options. These patients have especially poor outcomes when treated with chemo-immunotherapy, hence therapies like FCR are not chosen preferentially in them. Although age is not a deciding factor in the selection of the said options, young and fit patients have the option of hematopoietic stem cell transplantation, which may provide complete cure with but has the risk of transplant related mortality and morbidity.

Older patients:

To summarize, right off the bat, ibrutinib is the best option for the initial therapy of any patient aged 70 years or more, the caveat being the indefinite and often lifelong requirement of this drug. The second best option is venetoclax with obinutuzumab. That being said there are subpopulations of older patients who have options available with equal efficacy and which may prove useful in certain situations.

The data for use of ibrutinib in the first line come from a phase 3 study (Alliance A041202) in which patients 65 years of age or older who had untreated CLL were randomly assigned to receive bendamustine plus rituximab, ibrutinib, or ibrutinib plus rituximab. The primary endpoint was progression-free survival. Median progression-free survival was reached only with bendamustine plus rituximab. The estimated percentage of patients with progression-free survival at 2 years was 74% with bendamustine plus rituximab and was higher with ibrutinib alone (87%; hazard ratio for disease progression or death, 0.39; 95% confidence interval [CI], 0.26 to 0.58; P<0.001) and with ibrutinib plus rituximab (88%; hazard ratio, 0.38; 95% CI, 0.25 to

0.59; P<0.001). There was no significant difference between the ibrutinib-plus-rituximab group and the ibrutinib group with regard to progression-free survival (hazard ratio, 1.00; 95% CI, 0.62 to 1.62; P=0.49).

With a median follow-up of 38 months, there was no significant difference among the three treatment groups with regard to overall survival. The rate of grade 3, 4, or 5 hematologic adverse events were higher with bendamustine plus rituximab (61%) than with ibrutinib or ibrutinib plus rituximab (41% and 39%, respectively), whereas the rate of grade 3, 4, or 5 non hematologic adverse events were lower with bendamustine plus rituximab (63%) than with the ibrutinib-containing regimens (74% with each regimen).

Like in younger patients, IGHV mutation status plays an important role in informed decision making. If IGHV is **un**mutated (and without deletion 17p/*TP53* mutation), ibrutinib as single agent or a combination of venetoclax plus obinutuzumab should be chosen rather than chemoimmunotherapy. Ventoclax plus obinutuzumab as a short course fixed duration strategy offers advantage over ibrutinib in just that sense: it's a limited duration course and in patients having comorbidities like atrial fibrillation, cardiac conditions and those who require anticoagulants like warfarin, ibrutinib should not be the first choice.

The data supporting venetoclax plus obinutuzumab come from a recent phase 3 trial (CLL 14), in which fixed-duration treatment with venetoclax and obinutuzumab in patients with previously untreated CLL and coexisting conditions was studied. Patients with a score of greater than 6 on the Cumulative Illness Rating Scale (scores range from 0 to 56, with higher scores indicating more impaired function of organ systems) or a calculated creatinine clearance of less than 70 ml per minute were randomly assigned to receive venetoclax-obinutuzumab or chlorambucil-obinutuzumab. The primary end point was investigator-assessed progression-free survival. After a median follow-up of 28.1 months, 30 primary end-point events (disease progression or death) had occurred in the venetoclax-obinutuzumab group and 77 had occurred in the chlorambucil-obinutuzumab group (hazard ratio, 0.35; 95% confidence interval [CI], 0.23 to 0.53; $P<0.001$). The Kaplan-Meier estimate of the percentage of patients with progression-free survival at 24 months was significantly higher in the venetoclax-obinutuzumab group than in the chlorambucil-obinutuzumab group: 88.2% (95% CI, 83.7 to 92.6) as compared with 64.1% (95% CI, 57.4 to 70.8). This benefit was also observed in patients with TP53 deletion, mutation, or both and in patients with unmutated immunoglobulin heavy-chain genes. Grade 3 or 4 neutropenia occurred in 52.8% of patients in the venetoclax-obinutuzumab group and in 48.1% of patients in the chlorambucil-obinutuzumab group, and grade 3 or 4 infections occurred in 17.5% and 15.0%, respectively. All-cause mortality was 9.3% in the venetoclax-obinutuzumab group and 7.9% in the chlorambucil-obinutuzumab group.

For older patients with IGHV-mutated status (and without deletion 17p/*TP53* mutation), options include ibrutinib as a single agent, single agent venetoclax, combination of venetoclax plus obinutuzumab and chemoimmunotherapy (most commonly used combination being bendamustine and rituximab). In patients with comorbidities like atrial fibrillation, cardiac disorders and those who are taking anticoagulants for whatever indication, ibrutinib will not be a good choice and other options should be given first consideration. BR is a unique option for IGHV-mutated older adults (of course, without deletion 17p/*TP53* mutation), as it's a limited duration treatment as opposed to lifelong therapy of ibrutinib, and it may result in cure. But it's certainly more toxic than the other two options and the overall clinical scenario should dictate the final choice of treatment. For the patients who request a limited duration of treatment, the short course combination therapy of venetoclax plus obinutuzumab is a good strategy.

Other options for older patients **without** deletion 17p or *TP53* mutation are chlorambucil based com-

binations and fludarabine based combination, although some other options are also there but
they are reserved for exceptional circumstances
and many a times used in resource poor settings.
Fludarabine based combinations are not

Del(17p) or *TP53* mutations:

The quintessential "high-risk" CLL patient is one
who has del 17p or *TP53* mutation. These abnormalities not only are markers of overall poor prognosis, but also are predictive of poor response to
therapy. The conventional chemoimmunotherapy
(rituximab based combinations) are ineffective to
a large extent and whatever clinical benefit is at-
tained is short-lived.

In the face of such grave risk status, it's a great new
of patients that many effective therapy options
are now available. At the same time it should be
stressed that while these newer therapies are phe-
nomenally better than the older options; the overall survival and progression free survival outcomes
of patients with high-risk abnormalities remain
poorer compared to those who do not harbour such
abnormalities.

Two options are most effective in these patients.
Ibrutinib and the combination of venetoclax plus
obinutuzumab. If it's not contraindicated, ibrutinib is considered a better option. In patients who

are unfit to receive ibrutinib, either due to age or comorbidities then combination of venetoclax plus obinutuzumab is preferred. In some patients with prohibitive morbidities or frailty, venetoclax alone may be used, omitting obinutuzumab. Some studies are now evaluating the role of combination of ibrutinib plus venetoclax, initial results are promising, but for the time being this novel combination can't be recommended for routine clinical use. Idelalisib is used in relapsed setting and in some countries it is even approved in the frontline setting but it is unnecessarily toxic with no obvious benefits over the aforementioned molecules.

Patients who have del 17p or *TP53* mutation and who are young and/or fit enough to tolerate a hematopoietic stem cell transplant (HSCT) procedure, should be considered for it. The rationale behind this approach is that, as we have already discussed, patients with these genetic abnormalities have poor prognosis even if they are started on the newer molecules. And in these patients, HSCT may offer long-term disease control and may even cure. The problem with HSCT is the dangerously high transplant related mortality and morbidity, all in the face of the availability of safe and very effective alternates.

CHAPTER 6: RESPONSE EVALUATION

Not only the response criteria should be adhered to with accuracy, the time frame is also very important. It is very important to remember that at least two months must pass between completion of therapy and evaluation of response in the patients who were on a therapy, the duration of which was fixed; for example, 6 cycles of FCR or BR.

But the situation gets tricky in patients who are on medicine, the duration of which is practically indefinite (like ibrutinib) or in those who are on some form of maintenance therapy. In these patients the clinician should wait for the patient to attain a maximal response. Maximal response is not an absolute term, it's relative and temporal. Let's suppose that the patients has been on ibrutinib for some time. In the initial few months we will see all parameters improve and the responses will get better and better, but then as the disease burden starts to disappear to a large extent, further improvements will be slow or absent. When such a time comes the patient is said to have achieved maximal response. Counting from this time onwards, two months should elapse and then evaluation is to be done to categorise the response. Some have suggested to use MRD status to guide evaluation timeline, but this is not widely practiced.

There are three components of response evaluation:

1. History and physical examination (including constitutional symptoms assessment)
2. Peripheral blood evaluation
3. Bone marrow examination

Response categories:

1. **Complete response:**

CR means that the peripheral blood lymphocytes (evaluated by blood and differential count) are

$<4 \times 10^9$/L **and** no significant lymphadenopathy by physical examination (although in clinical trials CT scanning of the areas of interest is often done) **and** no splenomegaly or hepatomegaly by physical examination (in trials CT is performed) **and** absence of disease-related constitutional symptoms **with** neutrophils $\geq 1.5 \times 10^9$/L, platelets $\geq 100 \times 10^9$/L **and** hemoglobin ≥ 11.0 g/dL.

In practice the above mentioned criteria are presently considered sufficient to document CR. In trials on the other hand, criteria like MRD assessment and bone marrow examination are often used. Patient may show all of the above mentioned criteria of complete response but on bone marrow examination may show nodular areas, which is known are nodular partial response, the nature of these nodular islands should be evaluated using immunohistochemistry.

Some patients may have persistent cytopenias related to therapy, who are otherwise fulfilling other criteria of CR. These are labelled as CR with incomplete marrow recovery. The bone marrow examination of these patients don't show any clonal cell infiltrates.

2. Partial remission:

There are two sets of parameters for determining response; group A includes lymph node status, liver/spleen size, constitutional symptoms and circulating lymphocyte count; whereas group B includes platelet count, hemoglobin and bone marrow status. At least 2 parameters of group A *and* 1 parameter of group B need to improve, if previously abnormal to identify as partial remission. If only 1 parameter of both groups A and B was abnormal before therapy, only 1 needs to improve. Constitutional symptoms persisting for > 1 month should be recorded.

The definitions of such "improvements" are clearly mentioned in the guidelines, which are: a decrease in the number of blood lymphocytes to 50% or less from the value before therapy, reduction in lymphadenopathy compared with baseline (by cross-sectional imaging scans in clinical trials or by palpation in general practice) as defined by a decrease in lymph node size by 50% or more in either the sum of the products of the same enlarged lymph nodes selected at baseline as assessed by imaging (an established number in clinical trials of lymph nodes has been up to 6) **and** the sum of longest diameters of the same enlarged lymph nodes selected at baseline as assessed by physical examination (an established number in clinical trials of lymph nodes has been a maximum of 6), no increase in any lymph node and no new enlarged lymph node (diameter ≥1.5 cm). For small lymph nodes (longest diameter <1.5 cm), an increase <25% is not considered significant, a regression ≥50% of the extent of enlargement of the spleen below the costal margin defined by palpation, or normalization in size. When assessed by CT, scan spleen size must have regressed by ≥50% in length beyond normal, a regression of ≥50% of the extent of enlargement of the liver below the costal margin defined by palpation, or normalization in size.

The blood count should show **either** platelet counts >100 × 109/L or 50% improvement over baseline or. Hb >11.0 g/dL or 50% improvement over baseline without red blood cell transfusions or erythropoietin support..

3. Progressive disease

Appearance of any new lesion such as enlarged lymph nodes (≥1.5 cm), splenomegaly, hepatomegaly, or other organ infiltrates or an increase by ≥50% in greatest determined diameter of any previous site (≥1.5 cm) constitutes progressive disease.If the spleen is not enlarged to begin with, then a 2 cm or more enlargement below the costal line indicates progression; the same holds true for the patients in whom splenomegaly was there but resolved with treatment. If the preexisting splenomegaly responded to treatment, but didn't normalise then a 50% or more increase over its previous measurement of enlargement below the costal margin means the disease has progressed.

An increase in the liver size of ≥50% of the extent enlargement of the liver below the costal margin defined by palpation, or the de novo appearance of hepatomegaly is a progressive disease parameter. Although it should be emphasized here that liver is notoriously difficult to evaluate for lymphoid involvement, as many other conditions

If the number of blood lymphocytes increases by 50% or more with at least $5 \times 10^9/L$ B lymphocytes progression is suspected. It is very important to note here that some newer drugs (especially ibrutinib) often increase the blood lymphocyte count early in the course and this doesn't imply progression, rather it's because of redistribution of lymphocytes to the peripheral blood due to the unique mode of action of these drugs.

Sometimes the disease progresses in the form of Richter's transformation, which is diagnosis pathologically established by lymph node biopsy. Persistent cytopenias that can be directly attributed to CLL and not to autoimmune processes or therapy may imply progression, although utmost caution should be exercised before making such a diagnosis. If the therapy of CLL has long been completed and cytopenia occurs at least 3 months after treatment and bone marrow shows infiltration with clonal CLL cells, it implies progression.

4. Stable disease

Stable disease is a diagnosis of exclusion. If the patient is not in CR or PR and is not showing progressive disease either then stable disease is the diagnosis. It should be noted that stable disease designation is not a desirable one and constitutes "treatment failure"; the only desirable categories of response are CR and PR.

5. Relapse and refractory disease:

If a patient is showing no response at all to the therapy (CR/PR), he is refractory. If the patient shows initial response, but that response is lost with six months of the last dose of therapy then also the disease is said to be refractory. On the other hand, if the disease showed initial response but loses that response **after** 6 months of the last therapy then it's known as relapsed disease.

6. Minimal residual disease

Conventional means of response evaluation using clinical examination, radiology, routine peripheral blood and morphological bone marrow evaluation. Studies done on patients of CLL who had achieved a CR, using techniques such as PCR, flow cytometry and NGS, showed that some patients had clonal B cells present despite having no morphological evidence of it upon other studies.

These tests have been clinically validated and their use is desirable but not compulsory. As a general rule, these tests should be employed when there is an agreed upon plan of action, in case MRD status comes back positive.

Another very important aspect of monitoring of treatment related toxicity and other complications that arise due to disease process itself. Complications like hepatitis B reactivation, infections, tumor lysis syndrome, hyperleukocytosis, hematological toxicity et cetera must be watched for with high index of suspicion and timely corrective and preventive measures must be taken.

CHAPTER 7:
HEMATOPOIETIC STEM
CELL TRANSPLANT

As is evident from our previous discussion, CLL is a highly heterogeneous disease. Some patients are expected to live for years without any treatment whatsoever while others may succumb despite the best available treatment. HSCT in CLL can be either auto or allo. Allogeneic HSCT may prove to be curative, whereas autologous can't; at the same time the obvious drawback of allogeneic transplant is the mortality frequently related with it. An important and particularly unsolved issue at hand is the relevance of data from the previous era. The drugs like ibrutinib and venetoclax plus obinutuzumab are recent inventions and the previous data comparing outcomes of chemotherapy alone versus HSCT are less reflective of the trend to modern era medicine.

As far as exclusion criteria are concerned, nothing is absolute. Age is often a decisive parameter, although there are no clear cut guidelines and individualisation is a must. For autologous HSCT and non-myeloablative allogeneic HSCT required age is 75 years or less. In case of myeloablative HSCT age criteria are more restricted with less than 55 years being the desired age. I would like to stress again that age criteria are flexible and overall clinical picture dictates the decision making more.

We can divide the topic of HSCT in CLL in two broad headings: treatment naive and relapsed/refractory cases. In can be said with certainty that in patients who have not taken any treatment of CLL previously, HSCT is not a wise choice as the modern day medicines are capable of producing long lasting responses. Whereas in patients who are relapsed/refractory, the data are ambiguous regarding the exact benefit of performing HSCT but one thing is clear that with each successive failed chemotherapy regimen the chances of attaining and sustaining a favorable response plummet, so HSCT may be a good choice in such patients; especially those who attain a complete response to the preparatory therapy for HSCT (not conditioning). There are some patients of CLL who undergo transformation (Richter's), in them HSCT is the best possible option as otherwise the survival remains dismal.

Elaborating all the details of the methodologies and data pertaining to HSCT in CLL is well beyond the scope of this book. It suffices to state here that of the two types of HSCT available, autologous can only hope to improve PFS with virtually no effect on OS whereas the allogeneic one may provide cure but with very high mortality rate, being nearly 50% for myeloablative conditioning and upto 25% for reduced intensity conditioning.

CHAPTER 8: RELAPSED/ REFRACTORY DISEASE

We have already discussed the criteria for diagnosing relapsed/refractory disease in the relevant section. One important consideration would be to evaluate for new development of genetic abnormalities like deletion 17p and *TP53* mutation. It is also important to note here that all patients with relapsed or refractory disease don't necessarily require treatment. The same criteria of selection of patients for treatment apply, as in treatment naive CLL.

Options of treatment are not dictated by a strict algorithmic approach, rather clinical factors, comorbidities, preferences of clinician and patient and, most importantly, the timing and type of previous therapy or therapies play a bigger role. Although idelalisib is not approved in the USA for first line treatment of CLL but in many European countries it is; point is that there are no drugs in the armamentarium against CLL which are exclusively for relapsed setting. So the choices are the same as for the initial treatment of CLL, and the order of preference and general principles also remain the same.

If the clinical factors permit and especially in refractory and those patients with a somewhat earlier relapse, ibrutinib is the most preferred agent. The data come from an RCT, RESONATE, in which ibrutinib significantly improved median PFS compared with ofatumumab (not reached versus 8.1 months, at a median follow up of 9.4 months). Overall survival was also significantly improved with ibrutinib with a hazard ratio of death being 0.43. Overall response rates were also significantly better. With the increasing experience with this drug, subsets are being identified which show resistance to ibrutinib, especially the C481S mutation.

The PI3K-delta inhibitor idelalisib in combination with rituximab is a good option for the relapsed and especially the refractory patients. Idelalisib has many unique toxicities and caution should be exercised.

Venetoclax is a BCL2 inhibitor, which has been approved in both frontline and relapsed/refractory settings in CLL. In the latter case, it has been approved in combination with rituximab. The patients should be started on a low dose and gradually escalated to the full dose of 400 mg daily, and after a week of this maximum dose rituximab is added. It has been approved in relapsed/refractory patients who have a deletion 17p/*TP53* mutation **and** have failed a B cell pathway inhibitor as well as in those patients who don't have such abnormalities regardless of previous lines of therapy.

Conventional chemotherapy molecules like fludarabine, pentostatin, bendamustine, chlorambucil et cetera are used frequently in R/R CLL in combination with anti-CD20 monoclonal antibodies. Monoclonal antibodies may be used alone for the treatment of CLL and so can be cytotoxic chemotherapy molecules. Other drugs which are less frequently used are alemtuzumab, lenalidomide, high dose steroids and the newer molecule under trials: acalabrutinib.

If the patient's medical condition permits, which is not very often the case with R/R CLL, HSCT is a viable option. That being said, it is imperative to consider the very high transplant related mortality, especially in R/R setting and the fact that the best results with HSCT are observed in those patients who are in remission before performing an HSCT.

www.ingramcontent.com/pod-product-compliance
Lightning Source LLC
Chambersburg PA
CBHW021912170526
45157CB00005B/2056